The Faith
to Free-Fall

DR. HEIDI PETAK

ISBN-10: 1502427761
ISBN-13: 978-1502427762

DEDICATION

For my Mama

CONTENTS

ACKNOWLEDGMENTS

Thank you to God
for making all things
BEAUTIFUL
in Your time,
to my husband, Brian,
for making me laugh,
to my four boys for your snuggles,
to my sister, Kimberly, for giving me
the faith to believe I can do anything,
to my Dad for your devotion to mom and my family,
to George & Nancy for your life-giving encouragement,
to Michalle, Joy, Lindsay, Kim, Martha & Carter
who let me dream and spurred me on,
and to my courageous friends
who inspired the writing
of this book:
Cindy Kreidel
Vanessa Williamson
Linda Greene
Sally Cleek
Michele Riley
Patty Seitz
Deborah Russell
Janet Moreno
Amanda Conley
Diana Pettit
Amy Dreier
Kristin Mullinix
Carla Risen

i

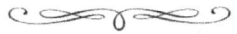

INTRODUCTION

My dear friend, I know you wish you weren't reading this right now. Because reading this means you are preparing to have a mastectomy. And that's a really tough pill to swallow. I'm with you! Mastectomies are things that happen to other people, right? Not you! Not me! Not us!

At this point, I imagine you are drowning in appointments, pamphlets and booklets, diagrams, statistics and options. You alternate between numb and crying, denying and terrified, incredulous that they could be talking about your body. I know, because I have been there. My heart is hurting for you as you read this, for the anguish, the grief, the fear you are undoubtedly experiencing.

Doctors are there to give you medical information and prepare you for what will happen to your body. But I know your spirit needs to be strengthened, too, as you wait for the big day. I needed it. And I know you need it.

I know what you don't need is a 300-page treatise on faith (you have enough to read already!), but I do know you need a breath of encouragement, of hope. Especially right before you go to sleep. For me, it's in the quiet moments after the sun goes down that I'm especially vulnerable to fear.

So, in the evenings before your surgery, may this little book be a place where you can curl up and read for a few minutes and then pray before you close your eyes for the night. And in doing so, may you find courage to face the days ahead.

In the end, my prayer is that the Lord will strengthen your spirit so that when you walk into that hospital, you will walk not in fear but in faith.

As much as my heart hurts for you, my heart also leaps for you, for the roots of trust that will be driven down deeper, the blooms that will surprise you, and the strong Arms that will catch you up as you free-fall into them.

With my love,

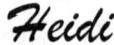

1

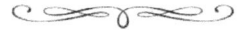

Shock

The doctor's lips move, announcing the news. You hear, but you don't hear. The words sear your ears and you shut out the noise, the news. Numb, you still have to walk. Out of the office, to the car.

You drive, numb. Stop lights blink colors, drivers mindlessly turn their wheels, yet how can the world keep on spinning when your world has stopped? You jab numbers, call family, choke out the facts.

Who am I talking about again? Not me. Really? Me?

Voices offer compassion, advice, even Scripture and prayers. But it's hard to take in. It's hard to feel anything at all. Except shocked.

Shock is our body's defense, our mind's compensation for a lightning strike. But the spirit, that core part of us where our emotions and character live, can't stay in denial for long. It wakes, blinks, incredulous exclamation, and then dives down again in hopes of waking to a different dream.

Pamphlets, percentages, decisions. The numbers and facts swirl like a tornado. Opinions, advice pummels, and your hands go to your head, overwhelmed. Shocked.

I know how you feel. You're not alone. I have been there. Millions of women before us have been there.

And in those moments when our spirit surfaces, we can't help but ask, "Where is God in all this?" Is He shocked, too? Hands to His divine head? Mouth open, incredulous?

I turn to Psalm 139:16, where David the Psalmist writes, "…in Your book were all written the days that were ordained for me, when as yet there was not one of them." God knows the number of our days before we were even born.

I read Isaiah 40:12 where God "measures the waters in the hollow of His hand and marks off the heavens by the span." Our God knows the number of drops in the seas and the inches of the sky.

He's the One who painstakingly fingers each star into place and spins Jupiter perfectly in its orbit. The One who draws the boundary of the tide and commands the morning sun to rise.

God isn't shocked.

Not only can He not be shocked, but He knows. And He *knew*.

Psalm 139 tells us that God is "intimately acquainted with all our ways," and that "even before a word is on our tongue," He knows what we are going to say. So when the doctor told you the news, God already knew what you would hear. And when you choked out the facts on the phone to your loved one, He already knew what you would say.

He isn't shocked, He knows, and He will carry you through this.

When I was shocked at my news, afraid of what lay ahead, my friend Karthi taught me to pray a breath prayer- a prayer that takes just a breath's time to pray. It was a prayer that came from the depths of my spirit, crying out to God.

My prayer was this: "Good Shepherd, carry me." It's the picture of a lamb on the shepherd's shoulders, being carried over rough terrain, through wolf-infested fields. That lamb was me. That lamb is you.

It's a prayer to pray not just once, but often. Every time the shock strikes your soul again. Every time the fear creeps in. Breathe. Pray.

Because the decision to entrust your journey to the Good Shepherd is a continual one.

So, right now, as you read this, let your spirit pray as you breathe out, "Good Shepherd, carry me." Breathe in. Breathe out, "Good Shepherd, carry me."

And if you let Him, He will.

I promise.

Prayer:

Good Shepherd, carry me. I don't have the strength to carry myself. Thank you that You aren't shocked. Thank You that You know, that You knew this news before I did. Thank You that You have gone before me and that You will go with me on this journey. I don't understand Your ways, but I know You are asking me to trust You. To trust You to carry me through tomorrow, the next day, the next week. You are my Good Shepherd and I need You. Please carry me. Amen.

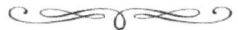

2

Anger

You lose your patience a little more quickly, snap at your loved ones a little more suddenly, slam the cupboard door a little harder.   And you feel it. Simmering deep within you.   Anger.

Anger that this is happening to you.   Anger that you can't do anything to stop it.   And maybe, just maybe, anger that God isn't doing anything to stop it.

Because the same divine Hand that spins Jupiter could just as easily reach down and pluck the cancer from your breast or change your genetic code, right?

Yes, He could.   Story after story in the Bible, from leprous Naaman to terminal Hezekiah, confirms that God has the power to miraculously heal.

We know that He can.

But often, He doesn't.

And that makes us mad.

Because we deserve to be healed, right?   Our pure and sinless life of devotion to God should be returned with a clean bill of health, right?

Weeellll, okay, so maybe we haven't been *completely* pure and sinless. Let's be honest.

My mind wanders back to the time as a teenager I bunched up my blanket to look like a sleeping person under the comforter on my bed and snuck out of my window to go mess around with my boyfriend.

Or the time years ago when I wasn't honest about the number of hours I had actually worked. Or when I didn't fess up to denting someone's car.

Or last week when I lost my patience and totally freaked out, yelling at my son for accidentally splattering orange fabric dye on my bathroom wall...

Okay, so maybe if I'm really honest, there's not much purity and a whole lot of sinfulness. I have a feeling you might come to the same conclusion after a glance back over your life.

But thank God for grace!   Grace that covers our sin through the blood of Jesus!   Otherwise, if it was about what we DESERVE, we should have all been struck by lightning the first time our little toddler mouths retorted, "No!"

But why this? Why me? Why now?

If we delve down really deep, peeling away layer after layer of emotion, of irritation, frustration, anger, what do you think we find at the bottom?

Fear.

Anger is actually a secondary emotion. There are two primary emotions that drive anger: hurt and fear. In this case, I believe the primary emotion is fear. We are afraid of what will happen to us. Afraid of the physical pain we will experience. Afraid for our family and the emotional pain they could experience. Afraid to die.

Your anger is normal. Your fear is normal. I felt it. I'm guessing we all feel it when we anticipate undergoing a mastectomy.

But it's what you do with your anger that will shape this journey for you.

Don't stuff it. Anger doesn't like to be stuffed. In fact, it rebels. Like an empty plastic bottle pushed down to the bottom of a sink of water, it keeps popping back up. And more often than not, it pops out sideways, smacking the people we love with hurtful words.

So feel what you need to feel. And face it head-on. Dive down deep to see what is under your anger, and ask God your hardest questions. God is a really big God. So big that our anger doesn't scare Him. Tell Him how you feel. He already knows anyway.

And when you are exhausted from pounding your fists into His chest, you will find His arms are wrapped around you, loving you unconditionally, even in your anger.

Prayer:

Lord, I'm mad. Mad this is happening and I can't stop it. And for some reason, You aren't stopping it. Thank You that You are big enough to handle my anger, and that You love me in the midst of it. You know I'm really just afraid. Afraid for my family, for my future, for my family's future. You promise that if I trust in You with all my heart and don't lean on my own understanding, You will direct my paths. I want to trust You. Please give me the courage and the faith to trust You more. Amen.

3

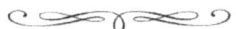

Fear

A thought, a word breaks through your anger and tears fall. Hot rivulets of fear. You reach for arms to hold you, to reassure you that everything is going to be okay.

Fear steals sleep, smothers peace and renders you immobile. The task of deciding dinner feels impossible. The mundane a stark contrast to the monumental.

In the days before my surgery, I had a zillion fears. And "experiencing pain" was at the top of the list. I have always dissolved into a puddle of tears merely anticipating having my blood drawn, so the idea of a major surgery was beyond my conception.

In fact, at a check-up last week the nurse exclaimed with her thick accent, "Ah remember you! You was the wimp from last yeeeah!" I laughed nervously and tried to erase the fear on my face as she prepped the needle

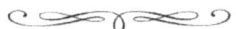

to draw my blood. I thought I looked brave until she said, "Hunny, you need to reee-lax. You look like you gonna pee on yo-self."

Thank you. Thank you very much. All that to say, during the days leading up to my mastectomy, I was sure it would be so painful I wouldn't be able to bear it.

But I did bear it.

Fear is just part of our human condition. That could very well be why the Bible has 365 verses that tell us to not be afraid! We need to be reminded every moment, every day of the year.

But our confidence doesn't rest in our ability to muster up courage. Our confidence rests in God, in His strength.

It's pure irony that His power is made perfect in weakness. I believe this irony is His design because when we are weak, we can't take any credit for strength.

So when we make it through another day, or when we make it through a major surgery, we have to thank Him for *His* grace, for *His* strength. And He gets the credit. Which is the way it should be.

You can trust that He will give you the strength you need to endure the next moment.

The next moment. You don't need strength to endure the next week, or the next month, or the next year. Just the next moment.

Corrie Ten Boom, a concentration camp survivor, wrote in her book, *The Hiding Place*, about the time she told her father she was afraid of losing him. He asked her, "When do I give you your train ticket?" She answered, "Just before I get on the train."

And so it is with us. We fear because we can't imagine having the strength to endure something like a mastectomy. But God gives us the strength we need at just the moment we need it.

God knows you're afraid. He sees you. He hears you. And He is with you. Even though I know it feels like a hurricane has swept into your life, you have a big God whose arms are tightly wrapped around you while the storm rages on.

Close your eyes and imagine that He is holding you. Hear the thunder, see the lightning, and feel His arms around you. Rest your head on His chest and listen to His heartbeat. His heart beats of His love for you, His care for you.

Claim this out loud from Psalm 56, "When I am afraid, I will put my trust in You, in God, whose word I praise. In God, I have put my trust."

A mastectomy may touch your body, but it can't touch your soul. Your soul is safe as you put your trust in Jesus Christ for your salvation and your future.

Prayer:

Heavenly Father, I'm afraid. I'm afraid of hospitals, doctors, needles. I'm afraid of pain. I don't want to go through this. And yet, You are asking me to trust You, to trust that You will give me the strength to endure whatever pain lies ahead. You promise in Philippians 4:8 that I can do all things through You because You give me strength. Please fill me with Your strength. I am choosing to give my fear to You tonight, to accept Your peace, and to rest. Amen.

Ten Boom, Corrie and Elizabeth and John Sherrill. *The Hiding Place*. Grand Rapids, MI: Chosen Books. 1984. 29. Print.

4

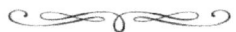

Honesty

A friend glances awkwardly at my chest and then back to my eyes. "How are you doing?" I shrug. "I'm okay." She asks, "Can I do anything for you?" I smile. "No. I'm fine."

I just lied. Twice.

Our temptation is to try to make things comfortable for others. We don't want them to feel awkward, so we cover our true feelings to make them easier to take. We don't want to put people out, so we don't let them in.

Or maybe we want to look stronger than we really are.

It takes humility to say what we really feel- to admit we're sad, we're hurting, we're scared, we're not strong. To admit we're weak and need help.

If you're a woman who likes to feel in control of your world (aren't we all?), it might be really hard to admit you need help. But maybe God is using this situation to help you surrender control, invite others in and trust Him more.

Our true friends, our loved ones - they want to be let in. To help with meals and dishes and hugs and comfort. They want to know what we need and how they can best support us. But often, they don't know what to do or how to do it. So they hang around, awkwardly silent, or they keep their distance, thinking that might be what we want.

My friend, Joy, wept, "I'm afraid I won't be a good friend to you through this." I assured her that just being with me was enough.

I did learn that I had to be very specific about what I needed. To not be specific is like sending someone to the grocery store without a list. You never know what you'll get! My husband loves to shop in bulk- so I know if I don't make a list we could end up with a year's supply of peanut butter in barrels that don't fit in the pantry.

So be specific. If you don't really know what you need, think about what encourages you most. Is it cards? Phone calls? Texts? People stopping by to give you an unexpected hug? People NOT stopping by? Would you like help around your house, people to play with your kids, or run an errand for you? Or maybe a friend to sit and talk over coffee, or go with you to buy a soft, button-up shirt to wear during your recovery?

When someone says, "Let me know if I can do anything for you," take her up on it! Ask a friend to organize a little prayer gathering, or maybe you would love it if your friends threw you a "pink party" to give you fuzzy socks and button-up shirts, or maybe you need a funny goodbye party for the "girls." Bravely ask a friend or family member to organize it.

If you're the default cook in your home, ask a friend or neighbor to set up a care calendar. She can email others in your neighborhood or workplace or church to sign up to bring a meal to your home during your recovery. You'll be very thankful for them.

People want to help. We just need to humble ourselves, admit we need help, and ask.

Another friend approaches me, asking, "Hey! I heard what you're going through. How are you doing?" I start to say my typical, "I'm okay," but decide to be honest. "It's really hard."

She hugs me. "I'm so sorry. Can I do anything for you?" Again, I'm tempted to answer with my usual "No, I'm fine." I don't want to seem needy.

But I remind myself that this is my friend, my friend God has given me for such a time as this. And she wants to help.

So, I decide to be honest. "I have a doctor's appointment tomorrow at 10 and I don't have anyone to watch my son. Could you possibly watch him?"

She nods eagerly, "Oh my goodness! Yes! Thanks for asking me. I can totally do that."

"Really, thank you! That would be great! Oh, also, Cindy's throwing me a little party Thursday night to pay our last respects to the 'girls,' if you wanna come."

She checks the calendar on her phone. "I want to come. Should I wear pink?"

"Pink…or black!"

"How about pink with black polka dots?"

"Perfect."

I'm thankful I was honest. Honesty builds trust- the core of relationships. And your relationships with your friends, your family, and your God will help you get through this- both before and after your surgery.

Prayer:

Lord, it's really hard to be honest. I want so much to look strong- I hate seeming needy. And yet You have put people in my life for such a time as this. When I do know what I need, please give me the courage and humility to be honest and ask for help. And when I don't know what I need, I pray that You will send the right people at just the right time to care for me. Thank You that You will provide for me through Your presence and through Your people. Amen.

5

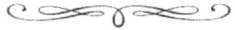

Grace

It's odd to have people looking at your chest. They ask questions, make comments, and place both of their feet firmly in their mouths…often.

One man asked me if I was afraid my surgery would affect my view of myself as a woman. I thought about asking him if castration would affect his perspective of his manhood, but bit my tongue instead and explained that my femininity goes way beyond body parts.

I suppose it's easier for me to have grace for other people when I know other people have had to have a lot of grace for me. I remember an acquaintance telling me she had undergone a mastectomy years earlier, however, my finite brain couldn't understand how she was still so shapely. So, I pointed to her breasts and asked, "Really? Then what are those?"

Not one of my finer moments. Obviously, I was clueless about the world of reconstruction.

So then, as various people said insensitive things to me in the days before my surgery, such as the well-meaning acquaintance who quipped, "I hope you're going to get some big kahunas out of this!," I tried to remember my vast capability at saying insensitive things. And so, I just laughed. If I could go back, I would add, "Yeah, that would be a perk, no pun intended."

Grace: Undeserved favor. It's what covers a multitude of sins- and a multitude of ill-chosen words, those of our friends and family as well as our own.

Don't ingest people's comments and let them fester anger and bitterness in your spirit. Grieve the hurt you may feel from what they said and then wrap the comments with grace and toss them heavenward. Then read the Word of God, take in what the Lord says to you and ingest it, letting *God's words* grow in your spirit, reaping joy and peace.

2 Corinthians 12:9 reminds us that God's grace is sufficient for us. It takes divine power to offer grace to others when you are feeling weak and afraid. But God's grace, poured out in buckets into our souls, cannot help but spill out onto the people around us.

In the coming days and weeks, you will have many opportunities to give grace to others, including grouchy nurses and edgy relatives, curious children and concerned neighbors. And because of the undeserved grace we have been given, we are able to offer grace to others. Yes, even those who, like us, don't deserve it.

Prayer:

Father, thank You for Your grace for me. I know I don't deserve it. And yet, You give me Your undeserved favor daily, freely, allowing me to live another day. I know people will say insensitive things to me in the coming weeks. (If anyone has said something insensitive to you already, tell God about it and how it made you feel. Physically act out wrapping up the comment and tossing it heavenward.) *I'm choosing to give their comments to You. As I respond to them, please help me to pour the same grace onto them that You have poured over and into me. I know I can't do it without You. Amen.*

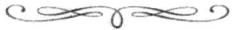

6

Sisterhood

You are about to join a sisterhood made up of millions of women who have had mastectomies before you. None of us would have volunteered to be in the club, but we are a part of it whether we like it or not.

There is an incredible family of support waiting, ready to help and love you through this season. Whether it's a support group or a website, or a friend or neighbor who has walked a similar road, I urge you to reach out and join the sisterhood.

In my neighborhood, like most neighborhoods, I know some folks better than others. Linda, my next-door neighbor, was one of the women I didn't know very well. We occasionally said hello to each other when we happened to arrive home at the same time or were out working in the yard, but didn't have much interaction aside from that.

However, the winter I was recovering from my surgery with my expanders still in my chest, I gave her family a tin of popcorn and our Christmas letter. In the letter I told my story about my surgery.

A few weeks later, another neighbor told me that Linda had been diagnosed with breast cancer and was facing a bilateral mastectomy.

Because I didn't know her well, I was hesitant to walk up and boldly knock on her door. So instead, I approached her husband as he was out getting the mail one day.

"Hi. I'm so sorry to hear the news about Linda. How is she doing?" He said she was having a tough time.

"I can imagine. Please tell her she's welcome to come talk to me anytime."

I found out later that Linda would go to the window and watch me playing with my kids outside. She longed to come out and talk but just couldn't bring herself to do it. She would muster up the courage, put on her coat and head to the door, only to crumple in tears before her hand touched the door handle. So she would take her coat back off again and retreat to weep alone in her bedroom.

Finally, one afternoon while I was playing catch with one of my sons, I looked up to see Linda crossing her yard towards mine. I smiled. "Linda! Hi!"

She smiled back, "Hi," but her sunglasses couldn't cover up her red, swollen eyes. And then, this woman and I who had cordially shared a yard for years, fell into each other's arms and cried.

There is nothing so beautiful and bonding as the sisterhood of women who face this surgery together.

After that big, initial step to walk out of her door and talk to me, Linda began to reach out to support groups as well and connect with other women who understood what she was feeling.

For the two of us, as we talked and prayed during those days and weeks before her surgery, we forged an unbreakable friendship.

It wasn't long after Linda returned home from the hospital that I knocked on her door again. She answered, grinning from ear to ear, her drains pinned to her waistband. To see my neighbor and friend smiling and full of hope gave me hope in my own journey.

And that's what we do in this sisterhood. We cry, we hug, we encourage, and we give each other hope.

Be courageous. Reach out. There's a wonderful family of women waiting, wanting to support you.

Welcome to the sisterhood.

Prayer:

Oh Lord, I never imagined I would be joining this sisterhood! And yet, this is a part of the story You are writing for me. Please give me the courage to make a phone call, to walk out of my door and share my heart with other women. And one day, I pray that You would give me the opportunity to be an encouragement to another woman who is walking this same road. Thank You for giving me the gift of community. Amen.

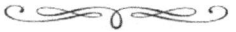

7

Grief

My counselor leans forward in her chair, "Heidi, you have to learn to lean into the pain."

What? Why would I want to do that? I would rather escape the pain. Take IB Profen, go shopping, eat chocolate, listen to music, watch TV, read interior decorating magazines.

"Lean into it" isn't on the list of what any of us naturally do when we experience pain. In fact, I think it sounds a little bit like volunteering for a root canal with no Novocain. No thank you.

But I'm learning. I'm learning to allow myself to feel all I need to feel. To not swallow away the lump in my throat but to let it get even lumpier. To not wipe away the tears but let them fall. (This stops with my nose, however. I will wipe it, thank you.)

Singer-songwriter Sarah Groves phrases her own revelation as, "I just showed up for my own life." I sing this line often to remind myself to really feel what I'm feeling.

When we allow ourselves to feel the emotional pain of anticipated loss, it's like we're pulling off the blinders and opening our eyes to see things for what they really are. And our spirit needs that revelation.

I have learned that when I stuff my feelings, trying to escape the pain, I suffocate my spirit and live gray. I believe color is found in the depths of our spirit, the richness of our emotions, and only when we take the plunge to see how deep the grief really goes can we truly live. In color.

And so, as you anticipate your surgery, give yourself the freedom to grieve, and to grieve deeply.

Our breasts have been with us our entire lives. Their development proclaimed our right of passage into womanhood. These life-giving glands have given us pleasure, fed our babies, and saggy as they might be, they are ours.

Saying goodbye to them is much more profound than saying goodbye to a suspicious mole or a problem kneecap. Our breasts are representative of our femininity and they have history. They're part of our story of being a woman.

How in the world, then, can we say goodbye to them?

Well, we say goodbye to them because we want to say hello to life. They've become a liability for living and so they have to go.

But they do need a proper send-off, a fitting goodbye for their many years of faithful service.

So, grieve their loss. Grieving will look different for each of us. And that's okay. For me, I needed to write. So I wrote an essay, a tribute to my "memory" glands. You can read it in the Epilogue at the end of this book.

I also wanted a goodbye ceremony with my husband. So, the night before my surgery, complete with music and dancing and all kinds of marital delights, we said goodbye. We celebrated, we prayed, we thanked, we cried- a lot. It was an essential part of my process.

It didn't make facing my surgery any easier, but it did help me feel the loss more fully, more deeply.

You might not want a goodbye ceremony. And if you do, your ceremony will probably look different from mine. And that's okay. Whatever you do, take the time to say goodbye in your own way.

It takes courage to truly grieve. In fact, it feels much better to escape. But when we're honest, leaning heavy into the pain of loss, we find that God is there.

In fact, He's the One we've been leaning into all along.

Prayer:

Father, You know all the things I typically do to escape pain. But I realize now You are asking me to resist escaping and to lean into You instead. Please help me to grieve fully, to give myself the freedom to feel all my emotions and not push them away. Thank You for the ability to truly feel. I want to lean on You, lean into You while I grieve. Please help me know and experience Your presence in the pain of this loss. Amen.

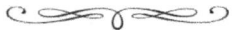

8

Beauty

"This one here is silicone and this one is saline," my plastic surgeon explains as he hands me two squishy breast implants.   It's surreal. I never, ever in a million years pictured myself sitting on an exam table fingering breast implants.

I'm ready to hand them back. "They're very…" what should I say? Interesting? Lifelike? I settle on "nice."

"They come in round, teardrop, smooth, textured. And I can do nipple reconstruction and then tattoo the areola."

Lovely. Can't wait for that. Wonder if I could get green areolas and gold nipples since my husband is a Packer fan?

"Would you like to see some pictures of my work?" he

asks. I'm not sure. Do I? Is this sort of like a dentist showing photos of his fillings or a car mechanic showing his refurbished carburetors?

I take the photos and flip through them. The pictures cut off the women at the neck and only show their breasts. I can hardly look at them. All I see are scars. My stomach turns. I close the album and hand it back to him.

My future. I just flipped through an album of my future. Will I ever be beautiful again?

If beauty is perfection, no. Then again, my droopy breasts that fed hungry babies aren't perfect now. And what is perfection, anyway? Is it not totally subjective? What might be beautiful in one culture isn't considered beautiful in another.

My mind drifts back a few years to the week I spent teaching women in South Sudan. Many of them had patterned tribal scars on their foreheads- considered beautiful to them and to the Sudanese men. Most assuredly, they sat bravely as the local sorcerer took the red-hot knife to their skin. This was their rite of passage, their celebration of beauty.

What if we could begin to anticipate our scars as a celebration of our beauty? Not a beauty defined by unblemished perfection, but a beauty of character. A beauty that shouts, "I chose life!"

Your scars will be beautiful symbols of your belief that

you have more to live for, that your life is worthwhile. To have no scars would mean that you crawled in bed and hid your head under the covers, hoping the cancer or the genetic mutation would go away. But if you have scars, it means you were proactive, courageous, and you believed in your own worth. You believed that God had more in store for you on this earth.

Proverbs 31:30 tells us, "Charm is deceitful and beauty is vain, but a woman who fears the Lord, she shall be praised."

It's not our unmarred skin that makes us beautiful. It's our character. Our character in choosing life and in trusting the Lord. While this journey is not at all the one we would have chosen for ourselves, this is the journey God allowed for us. And we must trust His goodness and His love.

A woman who walks in confidence, trusting in her God, beams hope and beauty. Not a skin-deep beauty, but a soul-deep beauty. And that's a beauty no surgeon can ever take away.

The nurse enters with a camera. "Alright, Heidi, we need to take some 'before' pictures."

Now, it's my turn. I swallow hard and take off my gown.

Today, my before and after pictures are in that photo album. I have scars. And I am beautiful.

Prayer:

Dear Lord, I know that in Your eyes, I'm beautiful. Not because of what I look like or what I've accomplished, but because I'm Your daughter, Your princess. Your banner over me is "LOVE," and because of Your love, I'm beautiful. You promise that You have good plans for me, plans to give me a hope and a future. I am clinging to You and to that hope tonight. Help me to one day see my scars as beautiful symbols that I chose life. Amen.

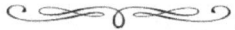

9

Gratitude

I was walking near a beach. The trail was lined with rocks pressed tightly together, sprinkled with hot, thirsty sand. Not a sprig of green was visible anywhere.

And then suddenly, I saw it. One yellow flower had courageously sprung up from between two rocks! "How crazy is that?" I thought. From where it got its nutrients I couldn't imagine, only that it must have driven its roots down deep to find them.

Some days it's really hard to have a positive attitude in the midst of the medical process of surgical preparation. I often felt like just a nameless body being poked and prodded. We know all of that is necessary, but our spirit, the core of who we are, feels a bit ignored.

"Wait!," we want to shout, "I'm not a statistic! I'm a real person with real feelings!" If we let ourselves, we can sink into depression, pessimism, hopelessness.

But what if we drive our roots down deep, believing that God is at work, that He is in control, and that He is writing our story? What if we looked for God-sightings, yellow flowers, glimpses of His grace in the midst of this hot, dry season?

The doctor who fit us in because of a last-minute cancellation, the tech who said an encouraging word, the empathetic glance of a loved one, the beautiful sunset, the hug of a child, the fuzzy, pink socks given to us by a friend... When we open our eyes to see the glimpses of God's grace, we begin to see them everywhere.

You might want to keep a gratitude journal, or just relay your grace-sightings to friends, family members, and medical staff.

Women who find things to be grateful for in this process stand out. In a landscape where many women are depressed, pessimistic and hopeless, gratitude might look at lot like a yellow flower springing up between rocks.

People may take a second look, wondering how your grateful attitude can even be possible. They might even ask you where in the world you're getting your strength to bloom.

The key is in making the choice to find things to be grateful for. Philippians 4:6-7 instructs you not to spend your time worrying, but to "pray about everything, to tell God your needs and don't forget to thank Him for His answers."

And then you're promised "if you do this, you will experience God's peace, which is far more wonderful than the human mind can understand. His peace will keep your thoughts and heart quiet and at rest as you trust in Christ Jesus" (TLB).

"Don't forget to thank Him for His answers." This is the phrase that precedes the gift of peace. His answers might be for things we didn't even pray for specifically, but perhaps someone else is praying those very things for us!

When we are anxious, feeling like a nameless body, worrying about our future, we need peace. And if gratitude leads to peace, I'm all in!

May gratitude sink your roots deep into faith in Jesus, believing that God is at work, that He is in control, and that He is writing your story. And then, may you rest in His peace- and bloom.

Prayer:

Oh Father, I need Your peace tonight. I keep feeling this fear creep back in when I think about the surgery and all of the details that have to fall into place while I'm in the hospital and while I recover. Whenever that fear creeps in, please help me to give it to You. Open my eyes to see glimpses of You and of Your grace all around me, and help me to be thankful. I want to shine for You, to bloom for You in this season, that others may ask where I'm getting my strength. And then I can tell them about You. I'm thankful for so many things tonight. (Now, tell Him everything you can think of!) *Thank You. Please cover me with Your peace. I rest in You. Amen.*

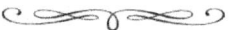

10

Free-Fall

Imagine sitting on the edge of the open door of a plane, 12,000 feet in the air, your heart racing, terrified. You feel the wind whipping wildly against your face, the roar of the plane engine so loud you can hardly think.

Someone near you yells, "You can't just fall out! The air pressure is too strong- you have to jump!"

Jump? That's crazy! That's a wild, crazy leap of faith!

You look down. This is it. You take a deep breath, bend your knees and…jump! Then…you're falling. Falling straight towards the earth, hurtling down at 120 miles per hour.

You squeeze your eyes tight and hold your breath as the wind rushes through your hair. This *is* crazy!

Slowly, you peek through the slits in your eyelids, and begin to breathe again. The sun is setting on the horizon, orange-red, blazing across the sky. Beautiful.

You take a deep breath and smile. All at once, the fear is gone. You lay flat on your back and stretch out your arms, floating, falling. It's suddenly quiet, still, like time has frozen. Total peace.

Most people would be terrified of free-falling, especially with no parachute. And for good reason! But you know how this spiritual free-fall ends.

You look down and see the earth, green, brown, spread out below you. Just a few more seconds to go. The earth rushes up to meet you, and then... instead of crashing into the hard ground, suddenly you are wrapped in warmth, in safety! You have fallen directly into the arms of Jesus. They're wrapped tightly around you. You're safe in His embrace.

My mom had a mastectomy in 2009. Later, she would describe being wheeled into the operating room as a "free-fall into the arms of Jesus." When I had my mastectomy one year later, I remembered her words as I was wheeled back. It did truly feel like a free-fall; all I could do was surrender my body and soul to God.

It takes faith to jump. It takes faith to free-fall.

And I know it's scary. Driving to the hospital the day of your surgery will take all of your willpower, all of your faith to keep heading that direction and not turn the car towards Tahiti.

But I also know there will be moments of peace that will surprise you. People God will send at just the right time with just the right words, verses of Scripture that will come to mind at just the moment you need them, supernatural strength He will give your loved ones to endure this journey with you.

God is writing your story. And your story isn't over yet. In fact, He might be just getting to the good part! Trust Him, believe Him, and jump. From there on out, it's a wild free-fall.

Whatever twists and turns your story takes, if you have put your faith in Jesus Christ for your salvation, I already know how your free-fall ends. Wrapped in His love, wrapped in His grace, and wrapped in His Arms.

That's me, that's you.

My dear friend, I'm giving you a hug tonight through these pages. My heart is with you.

Prayer:

Dear Lord, this is it! I'm about to jump out of the plane and free-fall. I need You. I can't do this without You. Please help me to believe You are writing my story and that my story ends well. I'm trusting You, trusting that Your strong Arms are waiting for me. Please give me the courage to jump, the strength to endure, and the faith to trust You. Amen.

EPILOGUE

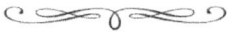

My Story

Three days before my mastectomy, I wrote an essay for a magazine contest. I didn't win the contest, but I'm thankful now that God gave me the incentive to write my story. I needed it. For my own mental, emotional and spiritual health- and for my heart. Here's the essay:

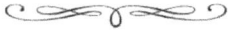

I hate goodbyes. No matter how many times I have had to say goodbye, it will always feel wrong and unnatural. Unless it's saying goodbye to a bad cold. I'm okay with that. Or an annoying solicitor. I'm okay with that, too.

But some goodbyes should never taint the odyssey of a life. My life.

41

On Wednesday, I have to say goodbye. Wednesday is less than three days from now- 57 hours, to be exact. All the atoms in my world are hurtling at light speed towards Wednesday. The day when I will walk into a hospital, allow an IV to be placed in my arm, and then surrender myself to sleep and to the waiting knife of a surgeon.

I hate needles, hospitals, pain, and goodbyes. Yet, I am choosing to say goodbye.

Last year, my mom was diagnosed with breast cancer. As she lay in bed recovering from a bilateral mastectomy, we began to unveil a family history riddled with breast and ovarian cancer. She was tested for a genetic mutation and her test came back positive for BRCA2. I was told that, as her daughter, there was a 50% chance that I carried the mutated gene as well. I decided to take the test.

Three weeks later, my husband and I returned to the doctor's office. We waited in the exam room, gripping each other's hand. The surgeon opened the door and walked in, holding a sheet of test results. "Well, you've got it!" he exclaimed, as if I had the winning number on a lottery ticket.

I was shocked, but I wasn't surprised. With my dark hair and brown eyes, I look exactly like my mother. It was fitting that I would share this element of her DNA as well.

The surgeon then explained that BRCA2 carries with it an up to 87% chance that I will be a victim of breast cancer in my lifetime. Since I'm "nipping" the heels of 40, he strongly recommended a bilateral mastectomy as soon as possible.

Say goodbye to my breasts? How could I do that? As a girl, I remember feeling the first thickening circles under my skin, signaling that I was becoming a woman. I remember my excitement when I wore my first bra, proud that I was finally "developing," as my mother called it. My breasts have since provided pleasure for me and my husband, fed four hungry babies, and played a leading role in the formation of my identity as a woman. How can I say goodbye to these "memory" glands?

After the shocking news, we drove into our driveway, greeted as usual by our four rambunctious boys, ages 7, 5, 3, and 1. They tackled me on the living room floor, giggling and wrestling like a heap of exuberant puppies. I love them.

I love the sparkling blue eyes of my oldest and the whimsical freckles that dot his cheeks. I love the passionate personality of my second-born that matches his wild red hair perfectly. I love the deep brown eyes and melt-in-your-mouth curls of my 3-year old, and how he tells me all about "Stai Wais" because he can't say his "r's" yet. And I love the unmatched smell of my baby's neck when he's fresh out of a Shea butter bath.

As much as I enjoy my breasts, I would choose my boys over my breasts without hesitation. I don't want to miss a minute of the richness of being their mommy.

And I don't want them to ever have to say goodbye to me.

Eighty-seven percent chance. If I were a betting woman, I would say that's a pretty good bet. And so, I have made the decision. The breasts have to go. They have become a liability, a time bomb ticking loudly, warning me that I need to decide what goodbyes I am willing to say. Given a choice, I will gladly say goodbye to two lumps on my chest to live to snuggle the four boys of my heart.

However, parting with something as significant as a body part, or two of them, demands a ceremony. That ceremony could either be a solemn occasion with candles and a eulogy, or it could be a raucous "pink party."

Twenty of my girlfriends opted for the raucous "pink party." Complete with a buxom bikini-top cake with "When Yours are Saggin,' She'll be Braggin," written in pink frosting, and armloads of thoughtful pink gifts, I was thoroughly showered with love and encouragement.

Three friends performed an original skit involving various types of fruit being stuffed in their shirts- from limes to pointy-stemmed pears and all sizes and textures of fruit in between. When the third woman grandly waltzed down the stairs with two watermelons in her shirt, we laughed until our faces hurt. They concluded their performance by singing, "You Lift Me Up" with revised lyrics.

After the gift-opening bonanza of soft pink socks, jammies, chocolate, books, tea, art supplies, and precious cards penned with kindness, they prayed over me with Scripture, songs, and words of comfort and strength. We cried until we couldn't cry any more. It was a fitting goodbye for my body parts.

Body parts. I don't like the sound of that. I know this will be painful, and I am far from courageous. I cry when I have to tweeze a splinter out of my hand. I don't want to experience pain- physical or emotional. I don't want to not be able to carry my little boys for six weeks, or weep because my baby won't be able to snuggle into my chest, hold my shirt and suck on his index finger like he loves to do.

But I do want to. Because I want to live. And so, I tearfully welcome Wednesday. I welcome the hospital and the IV, the knife and the pain. Because this goodbye isn't like any other. This goodbye just might grant me a longer lifetime of hellos.

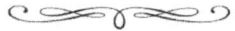

Those three days before my surgery flew by, and before I knew it, I was headed to the hospital. I arrived sad but hopeful, anxious but trusting, and ready to get it over with. My husband, Brian, and my friend, Cindy, who had been through a mastectomy before me, were at my side in the pre-op room. I distinctly remember Cindy's pink bandana as she read Scripture and prayed over me.

My recovery was long and tough, but God provided meals and support, care for my boys, friends who rubbed my feet and cleaned my fridge. Even people I hardly knew showed up to help! And by God's grace, I made it through.

However, I had no idea that the divine Author was about to add a new chapter to my story.

Five weeks after my surgery, while I was still on pain meds, my friend Vanessa approached me on the playground at church to tell me she had found a lump and was about to have a biopsy. She was soon diagnosed with breast cancer. As she anticipated her mastectomy, I poured back over Scripture, remembering the verses and thoughts that had given me the most comfort and shared them with her.

A crazy bunch of us threw her a pink party and I got to play a character in the fruit skit! The morning of her surgery, I found myself in the same hospital and the same waiting room where I had waited before my surgery, only this time I was the one wearing the pink bandana reading Scripture and praying over her before she was wheeled back.

A few weeks later, my heart sank when I learned that my next-door neighbor, Linda, had breast cancer. (See chapter titled "Sisterhood.") Again, I pulled out the verses and thoughts that had given me strength and passed them on to her. The morning of her mastectomy I found myself there again-- in the same hospital and in the same waiting room that had now become so familiar.

Then it was another neighbor, and then another friend, and since then, I have been honored to walk this journey with many friends.

Friends like you.

Because even though you and I may have never met, we too, are bonded in heart.

In the coming days, I pray that when your body is weak and broken, your spirit will be strong and soaring.

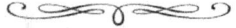

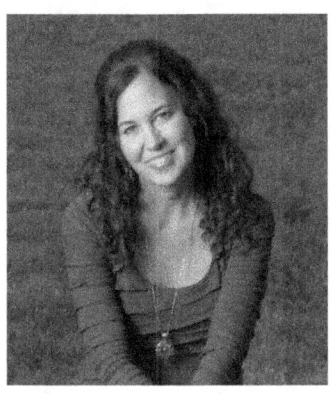

ABOUT THE AUTHOR

My kids will tell you I'm not the kind of doctor who looks in your ears. They're right. I'm actually a doctor of philosophy. I have a Ph.D. in communication and work as a communication coach, speaker, professor, voiceover artist and writer. My passion is to inspire others to communicate bravely in their professional and personal lives. For me, that includes communicating hope to those impacted by cancer or genetic mutations for cancer. I live in the Nashville area with my hubby, four boys, two birds, one fish, one cat, and one house rabbit named Louie.

Let's Connect!

Website/Blog: www.drheidipetak.com

Facebook: Dr. Heidi Petak   Twitter: @DrHeidiPetak

Instagram: drheidipetak   LinkedIn: Dr. Heidi Petak